METABOLIC CONFUSION MEAL PLAN FOR ENDOMORPH

A 28-Day Meal Plan to Boost Metabolism, Burn Fat, and Achieve Optimal Fitness with Easy Recipes, Carb Cycling Strategies, & Simple Exercise Guides

Andrew H. Steve

About the Author

Andrew H. Steve, a renowned nutrition and health expert, specializes in empowering individuals to reclaim their health. With a passion for nutrition and a deep understanding of the human body and metabolism, Andrew has successfully guided many to achieve significant weight loss and enhanced well-being.

With over a decade of experience, Andrew's approach is far from one-size-fits-all. He tailors his advice to each individual, focusing on a holistic method that encompasses a balanced diet, mindful eating, and an active lifestyle, rather than just diets and restrictions.

Known for his ability to distill complex dietary concepts into practical, actionable strategies, Andrew is a guiding force in navigating the intricacies of metabolism and wellness. His dedication extends beyond his professional achievements, as he finds joy in outdoor activities, experimenting with new recipes, and engaging in healthy discussions.

If you're looking to lose weight, increase energy, or improve your overall well-being, Andrew H. Steve is your ideal mentor. Under his guidance, you're not just adopting a healthy lifestyle; you're embarking on a transformative journey to rediscover your vitality and thrive.

TABLE OF CONTENTS

Chapter 1 6

Introduction to Metabolic Confusion Meal Plan 6

Understanding Metabolic Confusion 6

Endomorph Body Type 7

Chapter 2 9

Principles of the Metabolic Confusion Meal Plan 9

Metabolic Confusion Overview 9

Endomorph-Specific Considerations..........................11

Chapter 3 14

Nutritional Guidelines for Endomorphs 14

Macronutrient Ratios...14

Caloric Intake Recommendations 19

Timing of Meals and Snacks...................................23

Chapter 4 29

Meal Planning Strategies 29

Breakfast Recipes...29

Lunch Recipes 40

Dinner Recipes 50

Dessert Recipes 64

28 Days Sample Meal Plans.....................................75

Food Choices and Substitutions 83

Chapter 5 93

Metabolic Confusion Techniques 93

Calorie Cycling...93

Macronutrient Cycling 94

Intermittent Fasting Protocols 95

Chapter 6 98

Workout Integration..98

Importance of Exercise for Endomorphs.....................98

Matching Workouts with Meal Plans 101

Best Exercise Types for Endomorphs........................103

Chapter 7 112

Supplementation 112

Supplements to Support Metabolic Confusion 112

Timing and Dosage Recommendations 114

Chapter 8 116

Tracking Progress 116

Monitoring Body Composition Changes.....................116

Adjusting the Meal Plan Accordingly 118

Conclusion: Unleashing Your Metabolic Potential 120

Recap of Key Points 120

Long-Term Strategies for Metabolic Health................122

CHAPTER 1

INTRODUCTION TO METABOLIC CONFUSION MEAL PLAN

Welcome to a transformative journey towards unlocking the full potential of your metabolism through the Metabolic Confusion Meal Plan, specifically designed for individuals with the endomorphic body type. In this comprehensive guide, we delve deep into the realms of metabolic science, understanding the intricate dance between nutrition, exercise, and genetics, all while unravelling the mysteries of metabolic confusion.

Understanding Metabolic Confusion

At its core, metabolic confusion is a strategic approach to nutrition and exercise that aims to keep the body guessing and adaptively responding to stimuli, ultimately leading to enhanced metabolic flexibility and efficiency. The concept draws inspiration from the principles of muscle confusion in fitness training, where varied workouts prevent the body from plateauing and continuously adapting to new challenges.

Metabolic confusion embraces the dynamic nature of metabolism, recognizing that our bodies are incredibly adaptable and responsive to changes in diet and physical activity. By strategically cycling macronutrients, calories, and meal timing, we can disrupt the body's tendency to adapt to a specific routine, thereby stimulating metabolic processes and optimizing fat loss, muscle gain, and overall metabolic health.

Endomorph Body Type

Now, let's explore the unique characteristics of the endomorphic body type and how the Metabolic Confusion Meal Plan is tailored to address its specific needs. Endomorphs are often characterized by a higher percentage of body fat, a slower metabolic rate, and a propensity to store excess calories as fat.

However, it's essential to dispel the myth that being an endomorph equates to a predetermined fate of perpetual struggle with weight management. Instead, we embrace the inherent traits of endomorphs as a blueprint for crafting a personalized approach to nutrition and fitness that harnesses the power of metabolic confusion.

Endomorphs thrive on consistency and structure, yet they also benefit from variety and adaptability in their meal plans and workout routines. By strategically manipulating dietary variables such as calorie intake, macronutrient ratios, and meal timing, we can elicit profound changes in metabolic function, empowering endomorphs to achieve their fitness goals and unlock their full metabolic potential.

In the pages that follow, we embark on a holistic exploration of the Metabolic Confusion Meal Plan for endomorphs, encompassing nutritional guidelines, meal planning strategies, workout integration, supplementation, and tracking progress. Together, we will uncover the secrets to revitalizing your metabolism, transforming your body composition, and embracing a sustainable lifestyle rooted in metabolic health and vitality.

Get ready to embark on a journey of discovery, empowerment, and transformation as we dive into the world of metabolic confusion and unleash your metabolic potential like never before.

Let's embark on this journey together, and let the transformation begin.

CHAPTER 2

PRINCIPLES OF THE METABOLIC CONFUSION MEAL PLAN

In this chapter, we dive deep into the foundational principles of the Metabolic Confusion Meal Plan, exploring the intricacies of metabolic confusion and how it applies specifically to individuals with the endomorphic body type. From understanding the overarching philosophy behind metabolic confusion to delving into the unique considerations for endomorphs, we lay the groundwork for a transformative journey towards optimal metabolic health and fitness.

Metabolic Confusion Overview

Metabolic confusion is not merely a fad or a quick-fix solution but rather a strategic and scientifically grounded approach to nutrition and fitness. At its core, metabolic confusion revolves around the principle of keeping the body guessing and adaptively responding to stimuli, thereby preventing adaptation and stagnation.

The human body is incredibly adaptive, constantly striving to maintain homeostasis in response to changes in diet, exercise, and environmental factors. When we adhere to a static and predictable routine, whether it's in our dietary habits or workout regimens, our bodies eventually adapt to the stimuli, resulting in diminished returns in terms of metabolic efficiency and progress towards our fitness goals.

This is where metabolic confusion comes into play. By strategically introducing variations in key dietary variables such as calorie intake, macronutrient ratios, and meal timing, we disrupt the body's adaptive mechanisms, keeping it in a state of flux and prompting it to continually adapt and respond. This dynamic approach not only enhances metabolic flexibility but also accelerates fat loss, muscle gain, and overall metabolic health.

Metabolic confusion encompasses a variety of strategies and techniques, including calorie cycling, macronutrient cycling, and intermittent fasting protocols, each designed to elicit specific metabolic responses and optimize overall results. By incorporating these principles into our meal plan, we unlock the full potential of our metabolism and pave the way for sustainable long-term success.

Endomorph-Specific Considerations

As we delve deeper into the Metabolic Confusion Meal Plan, it's crucial to tailor our approach to the unique characteristics and needs of individuals with the endomorphic body type. Endomorphs are characterized by a higher percentage of body fat, a slower metabolic rate, and a propensity to store excess calories as fat.

While these traits may present challenges, they also serve as a blueprint for crafting a personalized approach to nutrition and fitness that leverages the power of metabolic confusion. Endomorphs thrive on consistency and structure, yet they also benefit from variety and adaptability in their meal plans and workout routines.

When designing a Metabolic Confusion Meal Plan for endomorphs, several key considerations come into play:

1. **Caloric Intake**: Endomorphs typically have a lower tolerance for excess calories due to their slower metabolic rate. By strategically cycling caloric intake, we can prevent the body from entering a state of energy surplus and promote fat loss while preserving lean muscle mass.

2. **Macronutrient Ratios**: Endomorphs may benefit from a higher protein intake to support muscle

growth and repair while moderating carbohydrate and fat intake to manage energy balance and insulin sensitivity. By cycling macronutrient ratios, we can optimize nutrient partitioning and metabolic function.

3. **Meal Timing**: Endomorphs may experience fluctuations in hunger and satiety due to variations in metabolic rate and insulin sensitivity. By incorporating intermittent fasting protocols or adjusting meal timing to align with periods of increased metabolic activity, we can optimize nutrient absorption and utilization.

4. **Supplementation**: Endomorphs may have specific nutrient deficiencies or metabolic imbalances that can be addressed through targeted supplementation. By supplementing strategically, we can support metabolic health and enhance the effectiveness of the meal plan.

5. **Exercise Integration**: Endomorphs may benefit from a combination of resistance training and cardiovascular exercise to optimize metabolic function and body composition. By matching workouts with meal plans and incorporating variety

into exercise routines, we can maximize calorie expenditure and metabolic adaptation.

By addressing these endomorph-specific considerations within the framework of the Metabolic Confusion Meal Plan, we empower individuals to overcome genetic predispositions and achieve their fitness goals with confidence and efficacy. With a personalized approach rooted in metabolic science and tailored to individual needs, we unlock the full potential of our metabolism and pave the way for sustainable long-term success.

In the next chapters, we'll delve deeper into the practical application of these principles, exploring nutritional guidelines, meal planning strategies, workout integration, supplementation, and tracking progress. Together, we'll embark on a transformative journey towards optimal metabolic health and fitness, fuelled by the power of metabolic confusion and tailored to the unique needs of endomorphs.

Get ready to unleash your metabolic potential and redefine what's possible for your body and your health.

CHAPTER 3

NUTRITIONAL GUIDELINES FOR ENDOMORPHS

Nutrition serves as the cornerstone of any successful fitness journey, and for endomorphs, understanding how to fuel the body optimally is paramount. In this chapter, we explore the specific nutritional guidelines tailored to the endomorphic body type, encompassing macronutrient ratios, caloric intake recommendations, and the timing of meals and snacks. Let's dive in and unlock the secrets to maximizing metabolic efficiency and achieving your health and fitness goals.

Macronutrient Ratios

1. **Protein:** Protein is the building block of muscle tissue and plays a crucial role in supporting muscle growth and repair. Aim for a protein intake comprising around 25-30% of your total daily calories. Opt for lean protein sources such as chicken, turkey, fish, tofu, and legumes to support your muscle-building endeavors.

2. **Carbohydrates:** Carbohydrates provide the body with energy and are essential for fueling workouts and replenishing glycogen stores. Aim to consume

approximately 40-45% of your total daily calories from carbohydrates. Focus on complex carbohydrates such as whole grains, fruits, vegetables, and legumes to provide sustained energy levels and support metabolic health.

3. **Fats:** Healthy fats are vital for hormone production, brain function, and overall health. Aim to include approximately 25-30% of your total daily calories from fats. Focus on sources of unsaturated fats such as avocados, nuts, seeds, olive oil, and fatty fish to promote satiety and support cardiovascular health.

4. **Fiber:** Adequate fiber intake is essential for digestive health and satiety. Aim to include plenty of fiber-rich foods such as fruits, vegetables, whole grains, and legumes in your diet to support digestive regularity and keep you feeling full and satisfied.

5. **Water:** Hydration is key for optimal metabolic function and overall health. Aim to drink plenty of water throughout the day to stay hydrated and support metabolic processes.

6. **Saturated Fats:** While unsaturated fats are essential for overall health, it's also important to moderate intake of saturated fats. Aim to limit

saturated fats to less than 10% of your total daily calories to support heart health and lower cholesterol levels. Sources of saturated fats include red meat, full-fat dairy products, and certain oils like coconut and palm oil.

7. **Trans Fats:** Avoid trans fats as much as possible, as they are linked to an increased risk of heart disease and other health issues. Trans fats are commonly found in processed and fried foods, margarine, and commercially baked goods. Aim to minimize trans fat intake to less than 1% of your total daily calories.

8. **Omega-3 Fatty Acids:** Incorporate omega-3 fatty acids into your diet to support brain health, reduce inflammation, and lower the risk of chronic diseases. Aim to include sources of omega-3 fatty acids such as fatty fish (salmon, mackerel, sardines), flaxseeds, chia seeds, walnuts, and hemp seeds. Aim for a ratio of omega-6 to omega-3 fatty acids of around 2:1 to maintain optimal health.

9. **Monounsaturated Fats:** Monounsaturated fats are known for their heart-healthy benefits and can help lower bad cholesterol levels while increasing good cholesterol levels. Include sources of

monounsaturated fats such as avocados, olives, nuts, and olive oil in your diet. Aim for monounsaturated fats to comprise around 15-20% of your total daily calories.

10. **Polyunsaturated Fats:** Polyunsaturated fats are essential fats that the body cannot produce on its own and must be obtained from food sources. Include sources of polyunsaturated fats such as sunflower seeds, pumpkin seeds, soybean oil, and fatty fish in your diet. Aim for polyunsaturated fats to comprise around 10-15% of your total daily calories.

11. **Simple Carbohydrates:** While complex carbohydrates are preferred for sustained energy levels, there may be times when simple carbohydrates are appropriate, such as during intense workouts or post-workout recovery. Aim to include simple carbohydrates from sources like fruits, honey, and sports drinks strategically to replenish glycogen stores and support recovery.

12. **Net Carbohydrates:** Net carbohydrates represent the total carbohydrates in a food minus the fiber content. Focus on net carbohydrates when tracking your carbohydrate intake, especially if you're

following a low-carb or ketogenic diet. Aim to include fiber-rich foods to minimize the impact of net carbohydrates on blood sugar levels and support digestive health.

13. **Glycemic Index:** Consider the glycemic index (GI) of carbohydrates when planning your meals. Foods with a low GI are digested and absorbed more slowly, resulting in gradual increases in blood sugar levels and sustained energy levels. Aim to include low GI carbohydrates such as whole grains, legumes, and non-starchy vegetables to support stable blood sugar levels and sustained energy.

14. **Timing of Carbohydrates: Pay** attention to the timing of your carbohydrate intake, especially around workouts. Consuming carbohydrates before and after exercise can help fuel workouts, replenish glycogen stores, and support muscle recovery. Aim to include carbohydrates in your pre-workout and post-workout meals or snacks for optimal performance and recovery.

15. **Protein Quality:** Consider the quality of protein sources when planning your meals. Aim to include high-quality protein sources that provide all essential

amino acids necessary for muscle growth and repair. Choose lean protein sources such as poultry, fish, eggs, dairy, and plant-based sources like tofu and tempeh to support your muscle-building endeavors.

Caloric Intake Recommendations

1. **Basal Metabolic Rate (BMR):** Determine your basal metabolic rate, which is the number of calories your body needs to maintain basic physiological functions at rest. Various online calculators can help estimate your BMR based on factors such as age, gender, weight, height, and activity level.

2. **Total Daily Energy Expenditure (TDEE):** Calculate your total daily energy expenditure, which includes your BMR plus calories burned through physical activity. This gives you an estimate of the number of calories you need to maintain your current weight.

3. **Caloric Deficit:** To promote fat loss, aim to consume slightly fewer calories than your TDEE. A moderate caloric deficit of around 500-750 calories per day is generally recommended for sustainable weight loss without sacrificing muscle mass.

4. **Nutrient Density:** Focus on nutrient-dense foods that provide essential vitamins, minerals, and micronutrients while keeping calories in check. Prioritize whole, minimally processed foods to support overall health and well-being.

5. **Meal Frequency:** Experiment with meal frequency to find what works best for you. Some individuals may prefer three larger meals per day, while others may thrive on smaller, more frequent meals and snacks. Listen to your body's hunger and fullness cues to determine your ideal meal frequency.

6. **Hydration:** Remember to include fluids in your caloric intake considerations. Adequate hydration is essential for overall health and can also support weight management by promoting satiety and aiding in digestion. Aim to drink at least 8-10 cups of water per day, adjusting for factors such as activity level and climate.

7. **Protein Intake:** Ensure that your caloric intake includes an adequate amount of protein to support muscle maintenance, repair, and growth. Aim for approximately 0.8-1 gram of protein per kilogram of

body weight per day, adjusting based on activity level and fitness goals.

8. **Carbohydrate Timing:** Consider timing your carbohydrate intake around periods of increased activity, such as before and after workouts. This can help optimize energy levels and replenish glycogen stores, supporting performance and recovery.

9. **Balanced Meals:** Aim to create balanced meals that include a combination of protein, carbohydrates, and fats. This not only provides a variety of nutrients but also helps promote satiety and stable blood sugar levels throughout the day.

10. **Mindful Eating:** Practice mindful eating by paying attention to hunger and fullness cues, as well as the sensory experience of eating. Avoid distractions such as television or smartphones during meals, and take the time to savor and enjoy your food.

11. **Portion Control:** Be mindful of portion sizes to avoid overeating. Use visual cues such as palm size for protein, fist size for carbohydrates, and thumb size for fats as a rough guide for portion sizes.

12. **Food Quality:** Focus on the quality of your calories rather than just the quantity. Choose whole, nutrient-dense foods over highly processed options to maximize nutritional value and support overall health.

13. **Consistency:** Aim for consistency in your caloric intake from day to day, as erratic eating patterns can disrupt metabolism and make it challenging to achieve weight management goals.

14. **Gradual Changes: If** making changes to your caloric intake, do so gradually to allow your body to adjust and minimize the risk of negative side effects such as metabolic slowdown or nutrient deficiencies.

15. **Individual Variability:** Keep in mind that caloric intake recommendations are highly individual and may vary based on factors such as metabolism, body composition, activity level, and genetics. Experimentation and self-awareness are key to finding the right balance for your unique needs and goals.

Timing of Meals and Snacks

1. **Breakfast:** Start your day with a balanced breakfast to kickstart your metabolism and provide sustained energy levels. Aim to include a combination of protein, carbohydrates, and healthy fats to keep you feeling full and satisfied until your next meal.

2. **Pre-Workout Nutrition:** Fuel your workouts with a pre-workout snack or meal containing a combination of carbohydrates and protein. This will provide the energy you need to power through your workout and support muscle repair and recovery.

3. **Post-Workout Nutrition:** After your workout, refuel your body with a post-workout meal or snack containing carbohydrates and protein to replenish glycogen stores and support muscle recovery. Aim to consume this meal within 30-60 minutes of completing your workout for optimal recovery.

4. **Snacks:** Incorporate healthy snacks between meals to keep hunger at bay and maintain energy levels throughout the day. Choose nutrient-dense options such as fruits, vegetables, nuts, Greek yogurt, or whole-grain crackers to satisfy cravings and support metabolic health.

5. **Dinner:** Enjoy a balanced dinner containing lean protein, complex carbohydrates, and healthy fats to satisfy hunger and support overnight recovery and repair. Aim to eat dinner at least two to three hours before bedtime to allow for proper digestion and optimize sleep quality

6. **Mid-Morning Snack:** Combat mid-morning hunger pangs with a nutritious snack to maintain energy levels and focus. Opt for a balanced snack such as a piece of fruit with a handful of almonds, or Greek yogurt with a drizzle of honey.

7. **Lunch:** Refuel your body midday with a satisfying lunch that includes a balance of protein, carbohydrates, and healthy fats. Incorporate lean protein sources such as grilled chicken or tofu, paired with complex carbohydrates like quinoa or sweet potatoes, and a side of mixed greens with avocado for healthy fats.

8. **Afternoon Snack:** Beat the afternoon slump with a nutrient-rich snack to keep you energized and focused until dinner. Choose options such as carrot sticks with hummus, a small handful of trail mix, or a

protein smoothie made with spinach, banana, and protein powder.

9. **Pre-Dinner Snack:** If dinner is still a few hours away, enjoy a light pre-dinner snack to tide you over without spoiling your appetite. Opt for a small portion of cottage cheese with pineapple, a slice of whole-grain toast with avocado, or a handful of cherry tomatoes with mozzarella cheese.

10. **Evening Snack:** Indulge in a satisfying evening snack that satisfies cravings while still aligning with your nutritional goals. Choose options such as air-popped popcorn sprinkled with nutritional yeast, a small bowl of Greek yogurt with berries, or a piece of dark chocolate paired with a few almonds.

11. **Pre-Bed Snack:** If you find yourself feeling hungry before bedtime, enjoy a small pre-bed snack that won't disrupt your sleep but provides a boost of nutrition. Consider options such as a slice of whole-grain toast with almond butter, a cup of herbal tea with a drizzle of honey, or a small bowl of cottage cheese with sliced banana.

12. **Hydration Throughout the Day:** Remember to stay hydrated throughout the day by sipping water

regularly. Aim to drink at least eight glasses of water daily, and consider incorporating hydrating options such as herbal teas, infused water with fresh fruits or herbs, or coconut water for electrolyte replenishment.

13. **Pre-Workout Hydration:** Prioritize hydration before your workout by drinking water or a sports drink to ensure optimal performance and prevent dehydration. Aim to consume fluids approximately 30 minutes before exercise to maintain hydration levels during your workout session.

14. **Post-Workout Hydration**: Rehydrate your body after exercise by drinking fluids to replenish fluids lost through sweat. Choose options such as water, coconut water, or a sports drink to restore electrolyte balance and support recovery.

15. **Evening Hydration:** Hydrate your body before bedtime by enjoying a soothing cup of herbal tea or a glass of warm milk to promote relaxation and prepare for restful sleep. Avoid caffeinated beverages close to bedtime to prevent sleep disturbances.

16. **Hydration During Meals:** Enhance digestion and nutrient absorption by sipping water or other hydrating beverages during meals. However, avoid excessive fluid intake, which can dilute stomach acid and impair digestion. Aim to drink small sips of water throughout your meal to support hydration without interfering with digestion.

17. **Hydration Upon Waking:** Kickstart your day by rehydrating your body with a glass of water or a hydrating beverage upon waking. This helps replenish fluids lost overnight and jumpstarts your metabolism for the day ahead.

18. **Hydration Before Meals:** Drink a glass of water or another hydrating beverage before meals to promote feelings of fullness and prevent overeating. This simple strategy can help you control portion sizes and support weight management goals.

19. **Hydration Between Alcoholic Beverages:** If you choose to consume alcoholic beverages, hydrate between drinks by alternating alcoholic beverages with water or other non-alcoholic options. This helps prevent dehydration and mitigates the negative

effects of alcohol on hydration levels and overall well-being.

20. **Hydration During Exercise:** Stay hydrated during exercise by drinking fluids regularly to replace fluids lost through sweat and prevent dehydration. Aim to sip water or a sports drink every 15-20 minutes during prolonged or intense exercise sessions to maintain hydration and optimize performance.

CHAPTER 4

MEAL PLANNING STRATEGIES

Breakfast Recipes

1. Protein-Packed Omelette

Ingredients:

- 2 large eggs
- ¼ cup diced bell peppers
- ¼ cup diced onions
- ¼ cup diced tomatoes
- ¼ cup chopped spinach
- Salt and pepper to taste
- 1 tsp olive oil

Instructions:

1. In a bowl, whisk together eggs, salt, and pepper.
2. Heat olive oil in a non-stick skillet over medium heat.
3. Add diced vegetables to the skillet and sauté until tender.

4. Pour whisked eggs over the vegetables in the skillet.

5. Cook until the edges start to set, then gently lift the edges with a spatula and tilt the skillet to let the uncooked eggs flow underneath.

6. Once the omelette is set, fold it in half and cook for another minute.

7. Serve hot with a side of whole-grain toast or avocado slices.

Nutritional Information (per serving):

- Calories: 250

- Protein: 17g

- Carbohydrates: 9g

- Fat: 16g

2. Greek Yogurt Parfait

Ingredients:

- ½ cup plain Greek yogurt

- ¼ cup mixed berries (strawberries, blueberries, raspberries)

- 1 tbsp honey or maple syrup (optional)

- 2 tbsp granola

- 1 tbsp chopped nuts (almonds, walnuts)

Instructions:

1. In a glass or bowl, layer Greek yogurt, mixed berries, and granola.

2. Drizzle with honey or maple syrup if desired.

3. Top with chopped nuts for added crunch.

4. Serve chilled.

Nutritional Information (per serving):

- Calories: 250

- Protein: 18g

- Carbohydrates: 30g

- Fat: 8g

3. Avocado Toast with Poached Eggs

Ingredients:

- 2 slices whole-grain bread

- 1 ripe avocado

- 2 large eggs

- Salt and pepper to taste

- Red pepper flakes (optional)

- 1 tsp olive oil

Instructions:

1. Toast the whole-grain bread slices until golden brown.

2. Mash the ripe avocado and spread it evenly on the toasted bread slices.

3. In a saucepan, bring water to a simmer and add a splash of vinegar.

4. Crack eggs into the simmering water and poach for 3-4 minutes until the whites are set but the yolks are still runny.

5. Remove the poached eggs from the water with a slotted spoon and place them on top of the avocado toast.

6. Season with salt, pepper, and red pepper flakes if desired.

7. Drizzle with olive oil and serve immediately.

Nutritional Information (per serving):

- Calories: 320

- Protein: 15g

- Carbohydrates: 24g

- Fat: 20g

4. Quinoa Breakfast Bowl

Ingredients:

- ½ cup cooked quinoa

- ¼ cup sliced strawberries

- ¼ cup blueberries

- 1 tbsp almond butter

- 1 tbsp honey or maple syrup

- 1 tbsp chia seeds

Instructions:

1. In a bowl, layer cooked quinoa, sliced strawberries, and blueberries.

2. Drizzle with almond butter and honey or maple syrup.

3. Sprinkle chia seeds on top for added nutrition.

4. Mix well before serving.

Nutritional Information (per serving):

- Calories: 280

- Protein: 8g

- Carbohydrates: 40g

- Fat: 10g

5. Veggie Breakfast Burrito

Ingredients:

- 2 large eggs

- 1 whole-grain tortilla

- ¼ cup black beans

- ¼ cup diced bell peppers

- ¼ cup diced onions

- ¼ cup chopped spinach

- ¼ cup salsa

- Salt and pepper to taste

- 1 tsp olive oil

Instructions:

1. In a bowl, whisk together eggs, salt, and pepper.

2. Heat olive oil in a non-stick skillet over medium heat.

3. Add diced vegetables to the skillet and sauté until tender.

4. Pour whisked eggs over the vegetables in the skillet and scramble until cooked through.

5. Warm the whole-grain tortilla in the skillet or microwave.

6. Spread black beans and scrambled eggs on the tortilla.

7. Top with salsa and roll into a burrito.

8. Serve warm.

Nutritional Information (per serving):

- Calories: 350

- Protein: 20g

- Carbohydrates: 35g

- Fat: 15g

6. Spinach and Feta Breakfast Wrap

Ingredients:

- 2 large eggs

- 1 whole-grain tortilla

- ¼ cup chopped spinach

- 2 tbsp crumbled feta cheese

- Salt and pepper to taste

- 1 tsp olive oil

Instructions:

1. In a bowl, whisk together eggs, salt, and pepper.

2. Heat olive oil in a non-stick skillet over medium heat.

3. Add chopped spinach to the skillet and sauté until wilted.

4. Pour whisked eggs over the spinach in the skillet and scramble until cooked through.

5. Warm the whole-grain tortilla in the skillet or microwave.

6. Spread scrambled eggs and crumbled feta cheese on the tortilla.

7. Roll into a wrap and serve warm.

Nutritional Information (per serving):

- Calories: 320

- Protein: 20g

- Carbohydrates: 20g

- Fat: 18g

7. Banana Nut Overnight Oats

Ingredients:

- 1/2 cup rolled oats

- 1/2 cup unsweetened almond milk

- 1/2 ripe banana, mashed

- 1 tbsp chopped nuts (almonds, walnuts)

- 1 tsp honey or maple syrup

- 1/2 tsp cinnamon

Instructions:

1. In a mason jar or bowl, combine rolled oats, almond milk, mashed banana, chopped nuts, honey or maple syrup, and cinnamon.

2. Stir well to combine all ingredients.

3. Cover and refrigerate overnight.

4. In the morning, give the overnight oats a good stir and enjoy cold or warmed up.

Nutritional Information (per serving):

- Calories: 280

- Protein: 8g

- Carbohydrates: 40g

- Fat: 10g

8. Green Smoothie Bowl

Ingredients:

- 1 cup spinach

- 1/2 ripe banana

- 1/4 cup frozen mixed berries

- 1/2 cup unsweetened almond milk

- 1 tbsp chia seeds

- 1 tbsp almond butter

- Optional toppings: sliced banana, berries, granola, coconut flakes

Instructions:

1. In a blender, combine spinach, banana, frozen mixed berries, almond milk, chia seeds, and almond butter.

2. Blend until smooth and creamy.

3. Pour the smoothie into a bowl.

4. Top with sliced banana, berries, granola, and coconut flakes if desired.

5. Serve immediately.

Nutritional Information (per serving):

- Calories: 300

- Protein: 8g

- Carbohydrates: 40g

- Fat: 12g

1. Turkey and Avocado Wrap

Ingredients:

- 1 whole-grain tortilla

- 3 oz sliced turkey breast

- 1/4 avocado, sliced

- 1/4 cup shredded lettuce

- 1/4 cup sliced tomatoes

- 1 tbsp hummus

- Salt and pepper to taste

Instructions:

1. Lay the whole-grain tortilla flat on a clean surface.

2. Spread hummus evenly over the tortilla.

3. Layer sliced turkey breast, avocado slices, shredded lettuce, and sliced tomatoes on top of the hummus.

4. Season with salt and pepper to taste.

5. Roll the tortilla tightly into a wrap.

6. Slice in half and serve.

Nutritional Information (per serving):

- Calories: 320

- Protein: 20g

- Carbohydrates: 30g

- Fat: 15g

2. Grilled Chicken Salad

Ingredients:

- 4 oz grilled chicken breast, sliced

- 2 cups mixed greens (spinach, arugula, lettuce)

- 1/4 cup cherry tomatoes, halved

- 1/4 cup sliced cucumbers

- 1/4 cup shredded carrots

- 1/4 avocado, diced

- 1 tbsp balsamic vinaigrette dressing

Instructions:

1. In a large bowl, combine mixed greens, cherry tomatoes, sliced cucumbers, shredded carrots, and diced avocado.

2. Top the salad with sliced grilled chicken breast.

3. Drizzle balsamic vinaigrette dressing over the salad.

4. Toss gently to combine all ingredients.

5. Serve immediately.

Nutritional Information (per serving):

- Calories: 280

- Protein: 25g

- Carbohydrates: 15g

- Fat: 12g

3. Quinoa and Black Bean Salad

Ingredients:

- ½ cup cooked quinoa

- ¼ cup black beans, drained and rinsed

- ¼ cup diced bell peppers (red, yellow, or green)

- ¼ cup diced red onions

- ¼ cup chopped cilantro

- ½ avocado, diced

- Juice of 1 lime

- Salt and pepper to taste

Instructions:

1. In a large bowl, combine cooked quinoa, black beans, diced bell peppers, diced red onions, chopped cilantro, and diced avocado.

2. Squeeze fresh lime juice over the salad.

3. Season with salt and pepper to taste.

4. Toss gently to combine all ingredients.

5. Serve chilled or at room temperature.

Nutritional Information (per serving):

- Calories: 320

- Protein: 10g

- Carbohydrates: 40g

- Fat: 15g

4. Veggie and Hummus Wrap

Ingredients:

- 1 whole-grain tortilla

- 2 tbsp hummus

- ¼ cup shredded lettuce

- ¼ cup sliced cucumbers

- ¼ cup shredded carrots

- ¼ cup diced tomatoes

- ¼ cup sliced bell peppers (red, yellow, or green)

Instructions:

1. Lay the whole-grain tortilla flat on a clean surface.

2. Spread hummus evenly over the tortilla.

3. Layer shredded lettuce, sliced cucumbers, shredded carrots, diced tomatoes, and sliced bell peppers on top of the hummus.

4. Roll the tortilla tightly into a wrap.

5. Slice in half and serve.

Nutritional Information (per serving):

- Calories: 250

- Protein: 8g

- Carbohydrates: 30g

- Fat: 10g

5. Salmon and Quinoa Bowl

Ingredients:

- 4 oz grilled or baked salmon fillet

- ½ cup cooked quinoa

- ¼ cup steamed broccoli florets

- ¼ cup diced bell peppers (red, yellow, or green)

- ¼ cup sliced carrots

- 1 tbsp sesame seeds

- Soy sauce or tamari for drizzling (optional)

Instructions:

1. In a bowl, layer cooked quinoa, steamed broccoli florets, diced bell peppers, sliced carrots, and grilled or baked salmon fillet.

2. Sprinkle sesame seeds on top for added crunch.

3. Drizzle with soy sauce or tamari if desired.

4. Serve warm.

Nutritional Information (per serving):

- Calories: 350

- Protein: 25g

- Carbohydrates: 30g

- Fat: 15g

6. Chickpea and Veggie Salad

Ingredients:

- ½ cup canned chickpeas, drained and rinsed

- 2 cups mixed greens (spinach, arugula, lettuce)

- ¼ cup cherry tomatoes, halved

- ¼ cup sliced cucumbers

- ¼ cup sliced red onions

- ¼ cup diced bell peppers (red, yellow, or green)

- 1/4 avocado, diced

- 1 tbsp olive oil

- Juice of 1 lemon

- Salt and pepper to taste

Instructions:

1. In a large bowl, combine chickpeas, mixed greens, cherry tomatoes, sliced cucumbers, sliced red onions, diced bell peppers, and diced avocado.

2. Drizzle olive oil and fresh lemon juice over the salad.

3. Season with salt and pepper to taste.

4. Toss gently to combine all ingredients.

5. Serve chilled or at room temperature.

Nutritional Information (per serving):

- Calories: 300

- Protein: 10g

- Carbohydrates: 30g

- Fat: 15g

7. Egg Salad Lettuce Wraps

Ingredients:

- 2 hard-boiled eggs, chopped

- 1/4 cup diced celery

- 1/4 cup diced red onions

- 1 tbsp Greek yogurt

- 1 tsp Dijon mustard

- Salt and pepper to taste

- 4 large lettuce leaves (such as romaine or butter lettuce)

Instructions:

1. In a bowl, combine chopped hard-boiled eggs, diced celery, diced red onions, Greek yogurt, and Dijon mustard.

2. Season with salt and pepper to taste.

3. Divide the egg salad mixture evenly among the large lettuce leaves.

4. Roll each lettuce leaf into a wrap.

5. Serve chilled.

Nutritional Information (per serving):

- Calories: 220

- Protein: 15g

- Carbohydrates: 5g

- Fat: 15g

8. Tofu Stir-Fry with Brown Rice

Ingredients:

- 4 oz firm tofu, cubed

- 1 cup cooked brown rice

- ½ cup mixed vegetables (bell peppers, broccoli, carrots, snap peas)

- 1 tbsp soy sauce or tamari

- 1 tsp sesame oil

- 1/2 tsp ginger, minced

- ½ tsp garlic, minced

- 1 green onion, sliced

Instructions:

1. Heat sesame oil in a skillet over medium heat.

2. Add minced ginger and garlic to the skillet and sauté until fragrant.

3. Add cubed tofu and cook until lightly browned on all sides.

4. Add mixed vegetables to the skillet and stir-fry until tender-crisp.

5. Stir in cooked brown rice and soy sauce or tamari.

6. Cook for an additional 2-3 minutes, stirring frequently.

7. Remove from heat and garnish with sliced green onions before serving.

Nutritional Information (per serving):

- Calories: 320

- Protein: 15g

- Carbohydrates: 40g

- Fat: 10g

Dinner Recipes

1. Baked Salmon with Roasted Vegetables

Ingredients:

- 4 oz salmon fillet

- 1 cup mixed vegetables (bell peppers, broccoli, carrots)

- 1 tbsp olive oil

- ½ tsp garlic powder

- ½ tsp paprika

- Salt and pepper to taste

- Lemon wedges for serving

Instructions:

1. Preheat the oven to 400°F (200°C).

2. Place the salmon fillet on a baking sheet lined with parchment paper.

3. In a bowl, toss the mixed vegetables with olive oil, garlic powder, paprika, salt, and pepper.

4. Spread the seasoned vegetables around the salmon on the baking sheet.

5. Bake in the preheated oven for 15-20 minutes or until the salmon is cooked through and the vegetables are tender.

6. Serve the baked salmon and roasted vegetables with lemon wedges.

Nutritional Information (per serving):

- Calories: 350

- Protein: 25g

- Carbohydrates: 15g

- Fat: 20g

2. Turkey and Quinoa Stuffed Bell Peppers

Ingredients:

- 2 large bell peppers

- ½ cup cooked quinoa

- 4 oz ground turkey

- ¼ cup diced tomatoes

- ¼ cup diced onions

- ¼ cup black beans, drained and rinsed

- ¼ cup shredded cheese

- 1 tsp olive oil

- Salt and pepper to taste

Instructions:

1. Preheat the oven to 375°F (190°C).

2. Cut the tops off the bell peppers and remove the seeds and membranes.

3. In a skillet, heat olive oil over medium heat and cook ground turkey until browned.

4. Add diced tomatoes, onions, and black beans to the skillet and cook until vegetables are tender.

5. Stir in cooked quinoa and season with salt and pepper.

6. Stuff the bell peppers with the turkey-quinoa mixture and place them in a baking dish.

7. Sprinkle shredded cheese on top of the stuffed bell peppers.

8. Bake in the preheated oven for 25-30 minutes or until the peppers are tender and the cheese is melted and bubbly.

9. Serve hot.

Nutritional Information (per serving):

- Calories: 320

- Protein: 25g

- Carbohydrates: 20g

- Fat: 15g

3. Chicken and Vegetable Stir-Fry

Ingredients:

- 4 oz chicken breast, sliced
- 1 cup mixed vegetables (bell peppers, broccoli, snap peas)
- 1 tbsp olive oil
- 2 tbsp soy sauce or tamari
- 1 tsp honey or maple syrup
- 1/2 tsp ginger, minced
- 1/2 tsp garlic, minced
- Sesame seeds for garnish
- Cooked brown rice for serving

Instructions:

1. In a bowl, whisk together soy sauce or tamari, honey or maple syrup, minced ginger, and minced garlic to make the stir-fry sauce.

2. Heat olive oil in a skillet over medium heat.

3. Add sliced chicken breast to the skillet and cook until browned and cooked through.

4. Add mixed vegetables to the skillet and stir-fry until tender-crisp.

5. Pour the stir-fry sauce over the chicken and vegetables in the skillet.

6. Cook for an additional 2-3 minutes, stirring frequently, until the sauce thickens and coats the chicken and vegetables.

7. Sprinkle sesame seeds on top for garnish.

8. Serve hot with cooked brown rice.

Nutritional Information (per serving):

- Calories: 350

- Protein: 25g

- Carbohydrates: 30g

- Fat: 15g

4. Lentil and Vegetable Curry

Ingredients:

- 1 cup cooked lentils

- 1 cup mixed vegetables (bell peppers, cauliflower, carrots)

- 1/2 cup diced tomatoes

- 1/2 cup coconut milk

- 1 tbsp curry powder

- 1 tsp olive oil

- Salt and pepper to taste

- Fresh cilantro for garnish

- Cooked quinoa or brown rice for serving

Instructions:

1. Heat olive oil in a skillet over medium heat.

2. Add mixed vegetables to the skillet and sauté until tender.

3. Stir in cooked lentils, diced tomatoes, coconut milk, and curry powder.

4. Season with salt and pepper to taste.

5. Simmer the curry mixture for 10-15 minutes, stirring occasionally, until heated through and vegetables are tender.

6. Serve hot with cooked quinoa or brown rice.

7. Garnish with fresh cilantro before serving.

Nutritional Information (per serving):

- Calories: 300

- Protein: 15g

- Carbohydrates: 35g

- Fat: 10g

5. Shrimp and Zucchini Noodles

Ingredients:

- 4 oz shrimp, peeled and deveined

- 1 large zucchini, spiralized into noodles

- ¼ cup diced tomatoes

- ¼ cup diced onions

- ¼ cup sliced bell peppers

- 1 clove garlic, minced

- 1 tbsp olive oil

- Juice of 1 lemon

- Salt and pepper to taste

- Fresh parsley for garnish

Instructions:

1. Heat olive oil in a skillet over medium heat.

2. Add minced garlic to the skillet and sauté until fragrant.

3. Add shrimp to the skillet and cook until pink and opaque.

4. Add diced tomatoes, onions, and sliced bell peppers to the skillet and cook until vegetables are tender.

5. Stir in spiralized zucchini noodles and lemon juice.

6. Season with salt and pepper to taste.

7. Cook for an additional 2-3 minutes, stirring frequently, until the zucchini noodles are heated through.

8. Serve hot with fresh parsley for garnish.

Nutritional Information (per serving):

- Calories: 250

- Protein: 20g

- Carbohydrates: 10g

- Fat: 10g

6. Tofu and Vegetable Stir-Fry

Ingredients:

- 4 oz firm tofu, cubed

- 1 cup mixed vegetables (bell peppers, broccoli, snap peas)

- 1 tbsp olive oil

- 2 tbsp soy sauce or tamari

- 1 tsp sesame oil

- ½ tsp ginger, minced

- 1/2 tsp garlic, minced

- Cooked quinoa or brown rice for serving

Instructions:

1. In a bowl, whisk together soy sauce or tamari, sesame oil, minced ginger, and minced garlic to make the stir-fry sauce.

2. Heat olive oil in a skillet over medium heat.

3. Add cubed tofu to the skillet and cook until lightly browned on all sides.

4. Add mixed vegetables to the skillet and stir-fry until tender-crisp.

5. Pour the stir-fry sauce over the tofu and vegetables in the skillet.

6. Cook for an additional 2-3 minutes, stirring frequently, until the sauce thickens and coats the tofu and vegetables.

7. Serve hot with cooked quinoa or brown rice.

Nutritional Information (per serving):

- Calories: 300

- Protein: 15g

- Carbohydrates: 25g

- Fat: 15g

7. Beef and Broccoli Stir-Fry

Ingredients:

- 4 oz beef sirloin, thinly sliced

- 1 cup broccoli florets

- ¼ cup sliced bell peppers

- 1/4 cup sliced onions

- 2 tbsp soy sauce or tamari

- 1 tsp olive oil

- ½ tsp ginger, minced

- ½ tsp garlic, minced

- Sesame seeds for garnish

- Cooked brown rice for serving

Instructions:

1. In a bowl, whisk together soy sauce or tamari, minced ginger, and minced garlic to make the stir-fry sauce.

2. Heat olive oil in a skillet over medium heat.

3. Add thinly sliced beef sirloin to the skillet and cook until browned.

4. Add broccoli florets, sliced bell peppers, and sliced onions to the skillet and stir-fry until tender-crisp.

5. Pour the stir-fry sauce over the beef and vegetables in the skillet.

6. Cook for an additional 2-3 minutes, stirring frequently, until the sauce thickens and coats the beef and vegetables.

7. Serve hot with cooked brown rice.

8. Garnish with sesame seeds before serving.

Nutritional Information (per serving):

- Calories: 350

- Protein: 25g

- Carbohydrates: 20g

- Fat: 18g

8. Eggplant and Chickpea Curry

Ingredients:

- 1 cup cooked chickpeas

- 1 medium eggplant, diced

- ½ cup diced tomatoes

- ¼ cup diced onions

- ¼ cup coconut milk

- 1 tbsp curry powder

- 1 tsp olive oil

- Salt and pepper to taste

- Fresh cilantro for garnish

- Cooked quinoa or brown rice for serving

Instructions:

1. Heat olive oil in a skillet over medium heat.

2. Add diced eggplant to the skillet and cook until softened.

3. Add diced tomatoes, onions, cooked chickpeas, coconut milk, and curry powder to the skillet.

4. Season with salt and pepper to taste.

5. Simmer the curry mixture for 10-15 minutes, stirring occasionally, until the eggplant is tender and the flavors are well combined.

6. Serve hot with cooked quinoa or brown rice.

7. Garnish with fresh cilantro before serving.

Nutritional Information (per serving):

- Calories: 320

- Protein: 10g

- Carbohydrates: 40g

- Fat: 15g

Dessert Recipes

1. Berry Protein Smoothie Bowl

Ingredients:

- ½ cup mixed berries (strawberries, blueberries, raspberries)

- ½ banana, frozen

- ½ cup plain Greek yogurt

- 1 scoop vanilla protein powder

- 1 tbsp almond butter

- 1 tbsp chia seeds

- Optional toppings: sliced strawberries, granola, coconut flakes

Instructions:

1. In a blender, combine mixed berries, frozen banana, Greek yogurt, vanilla protein powder, almond butter, and chia seeds.

2. Blend until smooth and creamy.

3. Pour the smoothie into a bowl.

4. Top with sliced strawberries, granola, and coconut flakes if desired.

5. Serve immediately.

Nutritional Information (per serving):

- Calories: 300

- Protein: 25g

- Carbohydrates: 30g

- Fat: 10g

2. Chocolate Avocado Mousse

Ingredients:

- 1 ripe avocado

- 2 tbsp unsweetened cocoa powder

- 3 tbsp honey or maple syrup

- ½ tsp vanilla extract

- Pinch of salt

- Fresh berries for garnish

Instructions:

1. In a blender or food processor, combine the ripe avocado, cocoa powder, honey or maple syrup, vanilla extract, and a pinch of salt.

2. Blend until smooth and creamy.

3. Spoon the chocolate avocado mousse into serving bowls.

4. Refrigerate for at least 30 minutes before serving.

5. Garnish with fresh berries before serving.

Nutritional Information (per serving):

- Calories: 220

- Protein: 3g

- Carbohydrates: 30g

- Fat: 12g

3. Greek Yogurt Parfait with Almond Crunch

Ingredients:

- ½ cup plain Greek yogurt

- ¼ cup mixed berries (strawberries, blueberries, raspberries)

- 2 tbsp granola

- 1 tbsp chopped almonds

- 1 tbsp honey or maple syrup

Instructions:

1. In a glass or bowl, layer Greek yogurt, mixed berries, granola, and chopped almonds.

2. Drizzle with honey or maple syrup.

3. Repeat the layers.

4. Serve chilled.

Nutritional Information (per serving):

- Calories: 250

- Protein: 15g

- Carbohydrates: 30g

- Fat: 10g

4. Peanut Butter Banana Protein Bites

Ingredients:

- 1 ripe banana, mashed

- ¼ cup natural peanut butter

- ½ cup rolled oats

- 1 scoop chocolate protein powder

- 1 tbsp honey or maple syrup

- ¼ cup dark chocolate chips

Instructions:

1. In a bowl, combine mashed banana, peanut butter, rolled oats, chocolate protein powder, honey or maple syrup, and dark chocolate chips.

2. Mix well until all ingredients are evenly incorporated.

3. Form the mixture into bite-sized balls.

4. Place the protein bites on a parchment-lined tray and refrigerate for at least 30 minutes.

5. Serve chilled.

Nutritional Information (per serving - 2 bites):

- Calories: 180

- Protein: 8g

- Carbohydrates: 20g

- Fat: 8g

5. Chia Seed Pudding with Mango

Ingredients:

- 2 tbsp chia seeds

- ½ cup unsweetened almond milk

- ½ tsp vanilla extract

- 1 tbsp honey or maple syrup

- ½ ripe mango, diced

- Fresh mint for garnish

Instructions:

1. In a bowl, mix chia seeds, almond milk, vanilla extract, and honey or maple syrup.

2. Stir well and refrigerate for at least 2 hours or overnight until the mixture thickens.

3. Spoon the chia pudding into serving glasses or bowls.

4. Top with diced mango and garnish with fresh mint.

5. Serve chilled.

Nutritional Information (per serving):

- Calories: 180

- Protein: 4g

- Carbohydrates: 25g

- Fat: 8g

6. Apple Cinnamon Baked Oatmeal Cups

Ingredients:

- 1 cup rolled oats

- ½ cup unsweetened applesauce

- ¼ cup almond milk

- 1 egg

- 1 tbsp honey or maple syrup

- 1 tsp cinnamon

- ½ tsp baking powder

- ¼ cup chopped nuts (walnuts or almonds)

Instructions:

1. Preheat the oven to 350°F (175°C) and grease a muffin tin.

2. In a bowl, mix rolled oats, applesauce, almond milk, egg, honey or maple syrup, cinnamon, and baking powder.

3. Divide the mixture evenly among the muffin cups.

4. Sprinkle chopped nuts on top.

5. Bake in the preheated oven for 20-25 minutes or until the tops are golden brown.

6. Allow the oatmeal cups to cool before removing them from the muffin tin.

7. Serve warm or at room temperature.

Nutritional Information (per serving - 2 oatmeal cups):

- Calories: 220

- Protein: 8g

- Carbohydrates: 30g

- Fat: 8g

7. Mixed Berry Yogurt Bark

Ingredients:

- 1 cup plain Greek yogurt

- ½ cup mixed berries (strawberries, blueberries, raspberries)

- 2 tbsp honey or maple syrup

- ¼ cup granola

Instructions:

1. Line a baking sheet with parchment paper.

2. In a bowl, mix Greek yogurt and honey or maple syrup until well combined.

3. Spread the yogurt mixture evenly onto the parchment paper.

4. Sprinkle mixed berries and granola on top of the yogurt.

5. Freeze for at least 2 hours or until firm.

6. Break the yogurt bark into pieces before serving.

Nutritional Information (per serving):

- Calories: 180

- Protein: 10g

- Carbohydrates: 25g

- Fat: 5g

8. Chocolate Protein Mug Cake

Ingredients:

- 1 scoop chocolate protein powder

- 1 tbsp almond flour

- 1 tbsp unsweetened cocoa powder

- ¼ tsp baking powder

- 1 egg

- 2 tbsp almond milk

- ½ tsp vanilla extract

- 1 tbsp dark chocolate chips

Instructions:

1. In a microwave-safe mug, mix chocolate protein powder, almond flour, cocoa powder, and baking powder.

2. Add egg, almond milk, and vanilla extract to the mug.

3. Mix until all ingredients are well combined.

4. Stir in dark chocolate chips.

5. Microwave on high for 1-2 minutes or until the cake is set.

6. Allow the mug cake to cool for a few minutes before serving.

Nutritional Information (per serving):

- Calories: 220

- Protein: 20g

- Carbohydrates: 15g

- Fat: 10g

28 Days Sample Meal Plans

Day 1:

- **Breakfast:** Berry Protein Smoothie Bowl
- **Lunch:** Grilled Chicken Salad
- **Dinner:** Baked Salmon with Roasted Vegetables
- **Dessert:** Apple Cinnamon Baked Oatmeal Cups

Day 2:

- Breakfast: Chocolate Avocado Mousse
- **Lunch:** Quinoa and Black Bean Salad
- **Dinner:** Tofu and Vegetable Stir-Fry
- **Dessert:** Mixed Berry Yogurt Bark

Day 3:

- **Breakfast:** Greek Yogurt Parfait with Almond Crunch
- **Lunch:** Chickpea and Veggie Salad
- **Dinner:** Beef and Broccoli Stir-Fry
- **Dessert:** Peanut Butter Banana Protein Bites

Day 4:

- **Breakfast:** Chia Seed Pudding with Mango
- **Lunch:** Veggie and Hummus Wrap
- **Dinner:** Lentil and Vegetable Curry
- **Dessert:** Chocolate Protein Mug Cake

Day 5:

- **Breakfast:** Peanut Butter Banana Smoothie
- **Lunch:** Turkey and Avocado Wrap
- **Dinner:** Shrimp and Zucchini Noodles
- **Dessert:** Mixed Berry Yogurt Bark

Day 6:

- **Breakfast:** Banana Berry Smoothie Bowl
- **Lunch:** Egg Salad Lettuce Wraps
- **Dinner:** Turkey and Quinoa Stuffed Bell Peppers
- **Dessert:** Apple Cinnamon Baked Oatmeal Cups

Day 7:

- **Breakfast:** Chocolate Protein Overnight Oats
- **Lunch:** Quinoa and Black Bean Salad

- **Dinner:** Beef and Broccoli Stir-Fry

- **Dessert:** Chocolate Avocado Mousse

Day 8:

- **Breakfast:** Mixed Berry Yogurt Parfait

- **Lunch:** Turkey and Avocado Wrap

- **Dinner:** Tofu and Vegetable Stir-Fry

- **Dessert:** Peanut Butter Banana Protein Bites

Day 9:

- **Breakfast:** Berry Protein Smoothie Bowl

- **Lunch:** Grilled Chicken Salad

- **Dinner:** Eggplant and Chickpea Curry

- **Dessert:** Mixed Berry Yogurt Bark

Day 10:

- **Breakfast:** Chocolate Avocado Mousse

- **Lunch:** Veggie and Hummus Wrap

- **Dinner:** Lentil and Vegetable Curry

- **Dessert:** Chocolate Protein Mug Cake

Day 11:

- **Breakfast:** Peanut Butter Banana Smoothie

- **Lunch:** Chickpea and Veggie Salad

- **Dinner:** Shrimp and Zucchini Noodles

- **Dessert:** Mixed Berry Yogurt Bark

Day 12:

- **Breakfast:** Banana Berry Smoothie Bowl

- **Lunch:** Egg Salad Lettuce Wraps

- **Dinner:** Turkey and Quinoa Stuffed Bell Peppers

- **Dessert:** Apple Cinnamon Baked Oatmeal Cups

Day 13:

- **Breakfast:** Chocolate Protein Overnight Oats

- **Lunch:** Quinoa and Black Bean Salad

- **Dinner:** Beef and Broccoli Stir-Fry

- **Dessert:** Chocolate Avocado Mousse

Day 14:

- **Breakfast:** Mixed Berry Yogurt Parfait

- **Lunch:** Turkey and Avocado Wrap

- **Dinner:** Tofu and Vegetable Stir-Fry

- **Dessert:** Peanut Butter Banana Protein Bites

Day 15:

- **Breakfast:** Berry Protein Smoothie Bowl

- **Lunch:** Grilled Chicken Salad

- **Dinner:** Baked Salmon with Roasted Vegetables

- **Dessert:** Apple Cinnamon Baked Oatmeal Cups

Day 16:

- **Breakfast:** Chocolate Avocado Mousse

- **Lunch:** Quinoa and Black Bean Salad

- **Dinner:** Tofu and Vegetable Stir-Fry

- **Dessert:** Mixed Berry Yogurt Bark

Day 17:

- **Breakfast:** Greek Yogurt Parfait with Almond Crunch

- **Lunch:** Chickpea and Veggie Salad

- **Dinner:** Beef and Broccoli Stir-Fry

- **Dessert:** Peanut Butter Banana Protein Bites

Day 18:

- **Breakfast:** Chia Seed Pudding with Mango
- **Lunch:** Veggie and Hummus Wrap
- **Dinner:** Lentil and Vegetable Curry
- **Dessert:** Chocolate Protein Mug Cake

Day 19:

- **Breakfast:** Peanut Butter Banana Smoothie
- **Lunch:** Turkey and Avocado Wrap
- **Dinner:** Shrimp and Zucchini Noodles
- **Dessert:** Mixed Berry Yogurt Bark

Day 20:

- **Breakfast:** Banana Berry Smoothie Bowl
- **Lunch:** Egg Salad Lettuce Wraps
- **Dinner:** Turkey and Quinoa Stuffed Bell Peppers
- **Dessert:** Apple Cinnamon Baked Oatmeal Cups

Day 21:

- **Breakfast:** Chocolate Protein Overnight Oats
- **Lunch:** Quinoa and Black Bean Salad

- **Dinner:** Beef and Broccoli Stir-Fry

- **Dessert:** Chocolate Avocado Mousse

Day 22:

- **Breakfast:** Mixed Berry Yogurt Parfait

- **Lunch:** Turkey and Avocado Wrap

- **Dinner:** Tofu and Vegetable Stir-Fry

- **Dessert:** Peanut Butter Banana Protein Bites

Day 23:

- **Breakfast:** Berry Protein Smoothie Bowl

- **Lunch:** Grilled Chicken Salad

- **Dinner:** Eggplant and Chickpea Curry

- **Dessert:** Mixed Berry Yogurt Bark

Day 24:

- **Breakfast:** Chocolate Avocado Mousse

- **Lunch:** Veggie and Hummus Wrap

- **Dinner:** Lentil and Vegetable Curry

- **Dessert:** Chocolate Protein Mug Cake

Day 25:

- **Breakfast:** Greek Yogurt Parfait with Almond Crunch

- **Lunch:** Chickpea and Veggie Salad

- **Dinner:** Shrimp and Zucchini Noodles

- **Dessert:** Apple Cinnamon Baked Oatmeal Cups

Day 26:

- **Breakfast:** Peanut Butter Banana Smoothie

- **Lunch:** Egg Salad Lettuce Wraps

- **Dinner:** Turkey and Quinoa Stuffed Bell Peppers

- **Dessert:** Mixed Berry Yogurt Bark

Day 27:

- **Breakfast:** Chocolate Protein Overnight Oats

- **Lunch:** Quinoa and Black Bean Salad

- **Dinner:** Beef and Broccoli Stir-Fry

- **Dessert:** Chocolate Avocado Mousse

Day 28:

- **Breakfast:** Mixed Berry Yogurt Parfait

- **Lunch:** Turkey and Avocado Wrap

- **Dinner:** Tofu and Vegetable Stir-Fry

- **Dessert:** Peanut Butter Banana Protein Bites

Food Choices and Substitutions

1. **Grains:**

   - Brown rice

   - Quinoa

   - Whole wheat pasta

   - Barley

   - Farro

   - **Substitutions:** Cauliflower rice, zucchini

   noodles (zoodles), bulgur wheat

2. **Proteins:**

   - Chicken breast

   - Salmon

   - Tofu

   - Lentils

- Turkey breast

- **Substitutions:** Lean beef, white fish (cod, tilapia), chickpeas, tempeh

3. **Vegetables:**

- Spinach

- Broccoli

- Bell peppers

- Kale

- Zucchini

- **Substitutions:** Swiss chard, Brussels sprouts, cauliflower, asparagus, collard greens

4. **Fruits:**

- Berries (strawberries, blueberries, raspberries)

- Bananas

- Apples

- Oranges

- Kiwi

- **Substitutions:** Mango, pineapple, grapes, peaches, pears

5. **Dairy:**

   - Greek yogurt

   - Cottage cheese

   - Feta cheese

   - Mozzarella cheese

   - Skim milk

   - **Substitutions:** Almond milk, coconut yogurt, tofu-based cheese, cashew cream

6. **Nuts and Seeds:**

   - Almonds

   - Walnuts

   - Chia seeds

   - Flaxseeds

   - Pumpkin seeds

   - **Substitutions:** Cashews, pecans, sunflower seeds, hemp seeds, sesame seeds

7. **Healthy Fats:**

- Avocado

- Olive oil

- Coconut oil

- Almond butter

- Flaxseed oil

- Substitutions: Peanut butter, tahini, sunflower oil, walnut oil, hemp oil

8. **Legumes:**

- Black beans

- Chickpeas

- Kidney beans

- Lentils

- Edamame

- **Substitutions:** Cannellini beans, navy beans, pinto beans, green peas, black-eyed peas

9. **Herbs and Spices:**

- Basil

- Cilantro

- Garlic

- Turmeric

- Cumin

- Substitutions: Parsley, rosemary, ginger, paprika, coriander

10. **Condiments:**

- Hummus

- Salsa

- Mustard

- Balsamic vinegar

- Soy sauce (low sodium)

- **Substitutions:** Guacamole, tahini sauce, hot sauce, apple cider vinegar, tamari sauce

11. **Whole Grains:**

- Oats

- Barley

- Bulgur

- Millet

- Whole wheat couscous

- **Substitutions:** Brown rice, quinoa, farro, buckwheat, amaranth

12. **Lean Proteins:**

    - Turkey breast

    - Chicken breast

    - White fish (cod, tilapia)

    - Lean beef (sirloin, tenderloin)

    - Egg whites

    - **Substitutions:** Tofu, tempeh, legumes (lentils, chickpeas), seitan, textured vegetable protein (TVP)

13. **Healthy Fats:**

    - Avocado

    - Olive oil

    - Coconut oil

- Nuts (almonds, walnuts)

- Seeds (chia seeds, flaxseeds)

- **Substitutions:** Nut butters (almond butter, peanut butter), seeds (sunflower seeds, pumpkin seeds), fatty fish (salmon, mackerel)

14. **Low-Glycemic Fruits:**

- Berries (strawberries, blueberries, raspberries)

- Apples

- Pears

- Cherries

- Grapefruit

- Substitutions: Kiwi, oranges, peaches, plums, apricots

15. **Leafy Greens:**

- Spinach

- Kale

- Swiss chard

- Collard greens

- Romaine lettuce

- **Substitutions:** Arugula, watercress, bok choy, mustard greens, beet greens

16. **Whole Grain Products:**

- Whole wheat bread

- Whole grain pasta

- Brown rice

- Quinoa

- Oats

- **Substitutions:** Spelt bread, buckwheat pasta, barley, farro, amaranth

17. **Lean Protein Sources:**

- Chicken breast

- Turkey breast

- White fish (cod, tilapia)

- Tofu

- Lentils

- **Substitutions:** Tempeh, seitan, edamame, chickpeas, legumes (black beans, kidney beans)

18. **Dairy Alternatives:**

- Almond milk

- Coconut yogurt

- Cashew cheese

- Soy milk

- Oat milk

- **Substitutions:** Rice milk, hemp milk, flax milk, coconut milk yogurt, almond-based cheese

19. **Healthy Snacks:**

- Greek yogurt with berries

- Hummus and vegetable sticks

- Apple slices with almond butter

- Mixed nuts

- Rice cakes with avocado

- **Substitutions:** Cottage cheese with fruit, guacamole with whole grain crackers, celery sticks with peanut butter, trail mix, whole grain toast with mashed banana

20. **Plant-Based Proteins:**

- Tofu

- Tempeh

- Seitan

- Lentils

- Chickpeas

- **Substitutions:** Edamame, textured vegetable protein (TVP), black beans, quinoa, hemp seeds

CHAPTER 5

METABOLIC CONFUSION TECHNIQUES

In this chapter, we delve into the transformative power of metabolic confusion techniques, exploring calorie cycling, macronutrient cycling, and intermittent fasting protocols. These strategies are essential components of the Metabolic Confusion Meal Plan, designed to keep your metabolism on its toes and maximize your body's adaptive response to dietary changes.

Calorie Cycling

Calorie cycling is a strategic approach to manipulating your daily calorie intake, alternating between periods of higher and lower calorie consumption. This technique capitalizes on the body's adaptive response to fluctuations in energy availability, preventing metabolic adaptation and promoting fat loss while preserving lean muscle mass.

Here's how calorie cycling works:

1. **High-Calorie Days**: On high-calorie days, you consume a surplus of calories, providing your body with ample energy to fuel workouts and support muscle growth. These days are typically aligned with

your most intense training sessions or days when you have higher energy demands.

2. **Low-Calorie Days**: Conversely, low-calorie days involve reducing your calorie intake below maintenance levels, creating a calorie deficit. This prompts your body to tap into stored fat for energy, facilitating fat loss while maintaining metabolic flexibility.

By alternating between high and low-calorie days, you prevent your metabolism from adapting to a consistent calorie intake, thereby optimizing fat loss, muscle gain, and overall metabolic health.

Macronutrient Cycling

Macronutrient cycling involves manipulating the ratio of carbohydrates, proteins, and fats in your diet on different days to optimize metabolic function and support your fitness goals. This technique leverages the varying metabolic responses elicited by different macronutrients, enhancing nutrient partitioning, insulin sensitivity, and metabolic flexibility.

Here's how macronutrient cycling works:

1. **High-Carb Days**: On high-carbohydrate days, you consume a greater proportion of your calories from carbohydrates, providing your body with readily available energy to fuel workouts and support glycogen replenishment. These days are typically aligned with intense training sessions or days when you have higher energy demands.

2. **Low-Carb Days**: Conversely, low-carbohydrate days involve reducing your carbohydrate intake and increasing your consumption of protein and healthy fats. This helps stabilize blood sugar levels, promote fat burning, and enhance satiety, making it easier to maintain a calorie deficit and support fat loss.

By cycling your macronutrient intake, you optimize nutrient timing and partitioning, enhance metabolic flexibility, and support your body's changing energy needs throughout the week.

Intermittent Fasting Protocols

Intermittent fasting (IF) is an eating pattern that alternates between periods of fasting and eating, cycling between periods of feeding and fasting to promote various metabolic benefits. IF protocols encompass several different fasting schedules, each with its unique approach to meal timing and frequency.

Here are some popular intermittent fasting protocols:

1. **16/8 Method**: This involves fasting for 16 hours each day and restricting your eating window to an 8-hour period. For example, you might skip breakfast and have your first meal at noon, followed by your last meal at 8 p.m. This protocol is often referred to as time-restricted feeding.

2. **Alternate-Day Fasting**: With this approach, you alternate between fasting days, where you consume minimal calories or fast completely, and feeding days, where you eat ad libitum. This protocol allows for more significant calorie restriction on fasting days, promoting fat loss while preserving lean muscle mass.

3. **5:2 Diet**: In this variation, you eat normally for five days of the week and restrict your calorie intake to 500-600 calories on two non-consecutive fasting days. This protocol provides a structured approach to intermittent fasting, making it easier to adhere to a calorie deficit while still enjoying regular meals on feeding days.

Intermittent fasting offers various metabolic benefits, including improved insulin sensitivity, enhanced autophagy, and increased fat oxidation. By incorporating intermittent fasting protocols into your meal plan, you can amplify the effects of calorie and macronutrient cycling, further optimizing your metabolic health and supporting your fitness goals.

CHAPTER 6

WORKOUT INTEGRATION

In this chapter, we delve into the crucial role of exercise in the Metabolic Confusion Meal Plan for endomorphs. We'll explore why exercise is essential for this body type, how to synchronize workouts with your meal plan for optimal results, and the best types of exercises specifically tailored to endomorphs.

Importance of Exercise for Endomorphs

Exercise isn't just about burning calories; it's a cornerstone of achieving metabolic balance and overall health, especially for endomorphs. Endomorphs tend to have a slower metabolic rate and a propensity to store excess calories as fat. Regular exercise helps counteract these tendencies by increasing metabolism, building lean muscle mass, and enhancing insulin sensitivity.

Moreover, exercise plays a crucial role in improving cardiovascular health, reducing the risk of chronic diseases, and boosting mood and mental well-being. For endomorphs, incorporating regular exercise into their routine is not just about aesthetics but also about optimizing metabolic function and overall health.

Here are 10 important exercises for endomorphs:

1. **Squats**: Squats are a compound lower-body exercise that targets the quadriceps, hamstrings, glutes, and core. They help build strength and muscle mass in the lower body, which can help endomorphs improve their metabolic rate and body composition.

2. **Deadlifts**: Deadlifts are another compound exercise that primarily targets the posterior chain muscles, including the hamstrings, glutes, and lower back. They are excellent for building overall strength and muscle mass, which is beneficial for endomorphs looking to increase their metabolism and burn fat.

3. **Lunges**: Lunges are a unilateral lower-body exercise that targets the quadriceps, hamstrings, glutes, and calves. They help improve balance, stability, and muscle coordination while also building strength and muscle mass in the lower body.

4. **Bench Press**: The bench press is a compound upper-body exercise that targets the chest,

shoulders, and triceps. It helps build upper-body strength and muscle mass, which is essential for endomorphs looking to improve their overall body composition.

5. **Pull-Ups/Chin-Ups**: Pull-ups and chin-ups are compound upper-body exercises that primarily target the back, biceps, and shoulders. They are excellent for building upper-body strength and muscle mass, which can help endomorphs increase their metabolism and burn fat.

6. **Rows**: Rows are a compound upper-body exercise that targets the back, biceps, and shoulders. They help improve upper-body strength, muscle mass, and posture, which is beneficial for endomorphs looking to improve their overall body composition.

7. **Planks**: Planks are an isometric core exercise that targets the abdominals, obliques, and lower back. They help improve core strength and stability, which is essential for maintaining proper posture and preventing injuries during other exercises.

8. **Russian Twists**: Russian twists are a core exercise that targets the obliques, abdominals, and lower back. They help improve rotational strength and

stability in the core, which is essential for functional movements and athletic performance.

9. **Mountain Climbers**: Mountain climbers are a dynamic core exercise that also engages the upper body and lower body. They help improve cardiovascular endurance, core strength, and coordination, making them an excellent addition to any endomorph's workout routine.

10. **HIIT (High-Intensity Interval Training)**: HIIT involves short bursts of high-intensity exercise followed by brief periods of rest or low-intensity recovery. It is highly effective for burning calories, improving cardiovascular fitness, and boosting metabolism, making it an ideal workout choice for endomorphs looking to maximize fat loss and metabolic efficiency.

Matching Workouts with Meal Plans

Synchronizing your workouts with your meal plan is key to maximizing the effectiveness of the Metabolic Confusion approach. The timing of your meals and exercise can influence your body's metabolic response, energy levels, and nutrient utilization. Here are some guidelines for matching workouts with meal plans:

1. **Pre-Workout Nutrition**: Fuel your workouts with a balanced meal or snack containing carbohydrates for energy and protein for muscle repair and growth. Timing your pre-workout meal 1-2 hours before exercise can optimize performance.

2. **Post-Workout Nutrition**: After exercise, refuel your body with a combination of protein and carbohydrates to replenish glycogen stores and support muscle recovery. Consuming a post-workout meal or snack within 30-60 minutes of exercise can enhance recovery and muscle protein synthesis.

3. **Meal Timing**: Structure your meals and snacks around your workouts to ensure adequate energy availability and nutrient intake. Consider your workout schedule when planning your meals to optimize performance and recovery.

By aligning your meal timing with your exercise routine, you can maximize the metabolic benefits of both and support your fitness goals more effectively.

Best Exercise Types for Endomorphs

When it comes to exercise, not all workouts are created equal, especially for endomorphs. Here are some of the best types of exercises tailored to the needs of endomorphs:

1. Strength Training: Strength training, also known as resistance training, forms the foundation of any effective workout routine for endomorphs. This type of exercise involves using resistance, such as weights, bands, or body weight, to build strength, muscle mass, and overall metabolic rate. Endomorphs benefit greatly from strength training due to its ability to increase lean muscle mass, which in turn boosts metabolism and improves body composition.

It's crucial for endomorphs to focus on compound exercises that engage multiple muscle groups simultaneously. These compound movements provide the most bang for your buck, allowing you to work multiple muscles in a single exercise. Examples of compound exercises include squats, deadlifts, lunges, and bench presses.

When incorporating strength training into your routine, aim for a mix of moderate to high-intensity sessions each week. This variety helps stimulate muscle growth and metabolic rate while preventing plateaus. Focus on progressively overloading your muscles by increasing the weight, reps, or sets over time to continue challenging your body and promoting growth.

2. High-Intensity Interval Training (HIIT): HIIT is a powerful tool for endomorphs looking to maximize fat loss and metabolic efficiency. This type of workout involves alternating between short bursts of high-intensity exercise and brief periods of rest or low-intensity recovery. HIIT workouts are highly effective at burning calories, improving cardiovascular fitness, and boosting metabolism.

For endomorphs, incorporating HIIT into their routine can help overcome plateaus and accelerate fat loss. HIIT workouts can be tailored to individual fitness levels and preferences, with exercises such as sprints, jumping jacks, burpees, or cycling sprints. The key is to push yourself to near-maximal effort during the high-intensity intervals, followed by active recovery periods to catch your breath and prepare for the next round.

HIIT workouts can be done in a relatively short amount of time, making them a convenient option for busy schedules. Aim to include HIIT sessions 2-3 times per week, alternating with strength training and other forms of exercise for a well-rounded fitness regimen.

3. Cardiovascular Exercise: While strength training and HIIT take precedence for endomorphs, cardiovascular exercise still plays a vital role in supporting overall health and weight management. Incorporating moderate-intensity cardio activities such as walking, jogging, cycling, or swimming into your routine can improve cardiovascular fitness, burn calories, and enhance recovery.

Cardiovascular exercise helps strengthen the heart and lungs, improves circulation, and boosts endurance, all of which are beneficial for overall health and well-being. Endomorphs can benefit from incorporating cardio sessions into their routine to complement their strength training and HIIT workouts.

Aim to include cardiovascular exercise 2-3 times per week, focusing on activities that you enjoy and can sustain for an extended period. Whether it's a brisk walk in nature, a leisurely bike ride, or a refreshing swim, find activities that you look forward to and can incorporate into your routine consistently.

4. Flexibility and Mobility Work: Flexibility and mobility exercises are often overlooked but are essential components of a well-rounded workout routine for endomorphs. These exercises focus on improving joint health, range of motion, and overall flexibility, reducing the risk of injuries and enhancing performance in other workouts.

Incorporating activities such as yoga, Pilates, or dynamic stretching into your routine can help improve flexibility, mobility, and overall movement quality. These exercises help release tension in tight muscles, improve posture, and enhance overall body awareness.

Aim to include flexibility and mobility work at least 2-3 times per week, either as standalone sessions or as part of your warm-up or cool-down routine. Focus on movements that target areas of tightness or stiffness, and remember to breathe deeply and mindfully as you move through each exercise.

5. Compound Movements with Isolation Variations: While compound exercises are excellent for targeting multiple muscle groups simultaneously, incorporating isolation variations can help endomorphs focus on specific muscle groups and improve muscle balance and symmetry. Examples include:

- **Leg Press**: Targets the quadriceps, hamstrings, and glutes with less stress on the lower back compared to squats.

- **Dumbbell Flyes**: Isolates the chest muscles, particularly the pectoralis major, providing a deep stretch and contraction for optimal muscle growth.

- **Hamstring Curls**: Isolates the hamstrings, helping to improve muscle tone and strength in the back of the legs.

By including compound movements alongside isolation variations, endomorphs can create a well-rounded strength training routine that addresses both overall muscle development and specific muscle groups.

6. Functional Training Exercises: Functional training focuses on movements that mimic real-life activities, improving overall movement patterns, stability, and mobility. Endomorphs can benefit from functional exercises that enhance everyday movements and reduce the risk of injury. Examples include:

- **Medicine Ball Slams**: Improves power and explosiveness while engaging the core, shoulders, and upper body.

- **Kettlebell Swings**: Targets the posterior chain muscles, including the hamstrings, glutes, and lower back, while also improving cardiovascular fitness.

- **Single-Leg Deadlifts**: Enhances balance, stability, and proprioception while targeting the hamstrings, glutes, and lower back.

Integrating functional training exercises into the workout routine helps endomorphs develop strength, stability, and mobility that translates into improved performance in daily activities and reduced risk of injury.

7. Stability and Balance Exercises: Stability and balance exercises are essential for improving proprioception, coordination, and joint stability, which are crucial for preventing injuries and enhancing overall athleticism. Endomorphs can benefit from stability and balance exercises such as:

- **Bosu Ball Squats**: Challenges balance and stability while targeting the lower body muscles, including the quadriceps, hamstrings, and glutes.

- **Single-Leg Balance Holds**: Improves balance and proprioception while engaging the stabilizing muscles of the lower body and core.

- **Plank Variations (Side Planks, Plank with Leg Lifts)**: Enhances core stability and strength while also engaging the shoulders, back, and glutes.

Incorporating stability and balance exercises into the workout routine helps endomorphs develop a strong foundation of stability and control, improving overall movement quality and reducing the risk of injury.

8. Plyometric Exercises: Plyometric exercises involve explosive movements that target fast-twitch muscle fibers, improving power, agility, and athletic performance. Endomorphs can incorporate plyometric exercises such as:

- **Box Jumps**: Improves lower body power and explosiveness while engaging the quadriceps, hamstrings, and glutes.

- **Jumping Lunges**: Enhances lower body strength and cardiovascular fitness while also improving coordination and agility.

- **Power Push-Ups**: Targets the chest, shoulders, and triceps while improving upper body power and explosiveness.

Including plyometric exercises in the workout routine helps endomorphs develop explosive strength and power, enhancing athletic performance and overall fitness.

9. Swimming: Swimming is an excellent low-impact cardiovascular exercise that engages the entire body, making it ideal for endomorphs looking to improve cardiovascular fitness without putting excessive strain on the joints. Swimming works the muscles of the arms, shoulders, back, core, and legs, providing a full-body workout that improves cardiovascular endurance and muscle tone.

Incorporating swimming into the workout routine offers a refreshing alternative to traditional cardio exercises while providing numerous benefits for overall health and fitness.

10. Circuit Training: Circuit training combines strength training and cardiovascular exercise into a single, efficient workout, making it an excellent option for endomorphs looking to maximize calorie burn and metabolic rate. Circuit training involves performing a series of exercises back-to-back with minimal rest in between, targeting different muscle groups and keeping the heart rate elevated throughout the workout.

CHAPTER 7

SUPPLEMENTATION

In our quest to optimize metabolic health and enhance the effectiveness of the Metabolic Confusion Meal Plan, supplementation emerges as a valuable tool. When used strategically and in conjunction with a balanced diet and regular exercise, supplements can complement our efforts, providing additional support for metabolic function, energy levels, and overall well-being. In this chapter, we explore the role of supplementation in supporting metabolic confusion, along with practical recommendations for timing and dosage.

Supplements to Support Metabolic Confusion

In addition to nutrition and exercise, certain supplements can complement the Metabolic Confusion Meal Plan and support metabolic optimization for endomorphs. While supplements are not a substitute for a balanced diet and regular exercise, they can enhance metabolic efficiency, promote fat loss, and support overall health when used strategically.

Here are some key supplements to consider incorporating into your regimen:

1. Protein Supplements: Protein powders or shakes can be convenient sources of high-quality protein to support muscle growth and repair, especially for individuals with higher protein requirements.

2. Branched-Chain Amino Acids (BCAAs): BCAAs, including leucine, isoleucine, and valine, are essential amino acids that play a crucial role in muscle protein synthesis and recovery. Supplementing with BCAAs can support muscle retention and reduce muscle breakdown during periods of calorie restriction.

3. Caffeine: Caffeine is a natural stimulant that can enhance energy levels, focus, and exercise performance. Consuming caffeine before workouts can increase calorie expenditure and fat oxidation, making it a valuable supplement for supporting fat loss.

4. Omega-3 Fatty Acids: Omega-3 fatty acids, found in fish oil supplements, have anti-inflammatory properties and support cardiovascular health. Supplementing with omega-3s can improve insulin sensitivity, reduce inflammation, and enhance fat metabolism.

5. Thermogenic Supplements: Certain supplements, such as green tea extract, capsaicin, and forskolin, have thermogenic properties that can increase metabolic rate and promote fat burning. However, it's essential to use these supplements cautiously and in moderation, as they can have side effects and interactions with other medications.

Timing and Dosage Recommendations

Optimal timing and dosage of supplements are essential considerations for maximizing their effectiveness and minimizing potential side effects. While individual needs may vary based on factors such as age, weight, activity level, and health status, here are some general guidelines for timing and dosage recommendations:

1. Protein Supplements: Consume protein supplements within 30 minutes to an hour post-workout to support muscle recovery and synthesis. Aim for a dosage of 20-30 grams of protein per serving, depending on your protein needs and meal timing.

2. BCAAs: Take BCAA supplements before, during, or after workouts to support muscle retention and reduce fatigue. A typical dosage ranges from 5 to 10 grams per serving, depending on your body weight and training intensity.

3. Caffeine: Consume caffeine supplements or beverages 30-60 minutes before workouts for optimal performance enhancement. Start with a lower dosage (e.g., 100-200 milligrams) to assess tolerance and gradually increase as needed, up to a maximum of 400 milligrams per day for most adults.

4. Omega-3 Fatty Acids: Take omega-3 supplements with meals to enhance absorption and minimize gastrointestinal discomfort. A standard dosage of fish oil supplements typically provides around 1,000-2,000 milligrams of combined EPA and DHA per day, although higher dosages may be recommended for specific health conditions.

5. Thermogenic Supplements: Follow the manufacturer's instructions for timing and dosage recommendations when taking thermogenic supplements. Start with the lowest effective dosage and monitor your response before increasing the dosage, and avoid consuming thermogenic supplements close to bedtime to prevent sleep disturbances.

CHAPTER 8

TRACKING PROGRESS

In our journey with the Metabolic Confusion Meal Plan for Endomorphs, tracking progress is not just about stepping on a scale or measuring inches. It's about understanding how your body responds to the dietary and lifestyle changes you've implemented, and using that information to make informed decisions moving forward. In this chapter, we'll explore two crucial aspects of tracking progress: monitoring body composition changes and adjusting the meal plan accordingly.

Monitoring Body Composition Changes

When it comes to tracking progress, focusing solely on weight can be misleading. Weight fluctuates due to various factors such as water retention, muscle gain, and hormonal fluctuations. Instead, it's essential to look beyond the scale and assess changes in body composition, which includes muscle mass, body fat percentage, and overall body shape.

1. Body Measurements: Take regular measurements of key areas such as waist, hips, thighs, and arms. These measurements can provide a more accurate representation of changes in body shape, especially when combined with progress photos.

2. Progress Photos: Visual progress is a powerful motivator. Take photos from multiple angles (front, side, and back) in consistent lighting and clothing to track changes in body composition over time.

3. Body Fat Percentage: Consider using methods such as skinfold calipers, bioelectrical impedance analysis (BIA), or DEXA scans to measure body fat percentage. While these methods may not be 100% accurate, they can still provide valuable insights into changes in lean mass and body fat.

4. Physical Performance: Pay attention to improvements in physical performance, such as increased strength, endurance, and mobility. These improvements indicate positive changes in muscle mass and overall fitness level.

5. Energy Levels and Well-being: Notice changes in energy levels, mood, and overall well-being. As your metabolism adjusts to the meal plan, you may experience changes in how you feel both physically and mentally.

Regularly tracking these aspects of body composition allows you to assess progress more comprehensively and adjust your approach as needed.

Adjusting the Meal Plan Accordingly

As you progress with the Metabolic Confusion Meal Plan, it's essential to remain flexible and adaptive. Your body's response to dietary changes may vary over time, requiring adjustments to keep your metabolism stimulated and your progress on track.

1. Assessing Progress: Review your tracking data regularly to assess how your body is responding to the meal plan. Look for trends and patterns in body composition changes, physical performance, and overall well-being.

2. Plateau Identification: If you notice a plateau in progress, where changes in body composition or physical performance stall despite adherence to the meal plan, it may be time to shake things up.

3. Calorie and Macronutrient Adjustments: Consider adjusting your calorie intake and macronutrient ratios based on your progress and goals. This may involve increasing or decreasing overall calorie intake, redistributing macronutrients, or experimenting with different meal timing strategies.

4. Meal Timing and Frequency: Evaluate your meal timing and frequency to ensure it aligns with your body's needs and preferences. Some endomorphs may benefit from more frequent, smaller meals, while others may thrive on intermittent fasting protocols.

5. Supplementation: Reassess your supplementation strategy to ensure it complements your evolving nutritional needs. Certain supplements, such as those supporting metabolism or muscle recovery, may become more or less relevant as your body composition changes.

6. Consultation with Professionals: If you're unsure how to adjust your meal plan or track progress effectively, consider consulting with a registered dietitian, nutritionist, or fitness coach. These professionals can provide personalized guidance based on your unique needs and goals.

Remember, progress is not always linear, and it's normal to experience ups and downs along the way. Stay patient, stay consistent, and trust the process as you continue on your journey with the Metabolic Confusion Meal Plan for Endomorphs.

CONCLUSION: UNLEASHING YOUR METABOLIC POTENTIAL

As we conclude our exploration of the Metabolic Confusion Meal Plan for Endomorphs, it's time to reflect on the key points we've covered and outline long-term strategies for maintaining metabolic health. Throughout this journey, we've delved into the intricacies of metabolic confusion, the unique characteristics of the endomorphic body type, and practical strategies for optimizing metabolic function. Now, let's recap the essential insights and discuss how to sustainably support metabolic health in the long run.

Recap of Key Points

1. Metabolic Confusion: We've learned that metabolic confusion is a strategic approach to nutrition and exercise, aimed at keeping the body adaptable and responsive to stimuli. By cycling macronutrients, calories, and meal timing, we disrupt the body's tendency to adapt to a specific routine, stimulating metabolic processes and optimizing fat loss, muscle gain, and overall metabolic health.

2. Endomorph Body Type: Endomorphs are characterized by a higher percentage of body fat, a slower metabolic rate, and a propensity to store excess calories as fat. However, we've debunked the myth that being an endomorph equates to a predetermined fate of perpetual struggle with weight management. Instead, we've embraced the inherent traits of endomorphs as a blueprint for crafting a personalized approach to nutrition and fitness that harnesses the power of metabolic confusion.

3. Meal Planning Strategies: We've explored meal planning strategies tailored specifically for endomorphs, including macronutrient ratios, calorie cycling, meal timing, and supplementation. By incorporating variety and adaptability into the meal plan, we've empowered endomorphs to optimize their metabolic health and achieve their fitness goals.

4. Tracking Progress: Tracking progress goes beyond simply measuring weight. We've emphasized the importance of monitoring body composition changes, physical performance, energy levels, and overall well-being. By regularly assessing progress, endomorphs can make informed adjustments to their meal plan and lifestyle to ensure continued success.

Long-Term Strategies for Metabolic Health

1. Lifestyle Sustainability: Sustainable lifestyle habits are key to long-term metabolic health. Endomorphs should focus on maintaining a balanced diet, regular physical activity, adequate sleep, stress management, and overall wellness practices.

2. Consistency and Adaptability: Consistency in following the principles of the Metabolic Confusion Meal Plan is essential for sustained metabolic health. However, it's also important to remain adaptable and open to making adjustments based on individual needs, goals, and progress.

3. Mindful Eating: Practicing mindful eating involves being aware of hunger cues, making conscious food choices, and savouring each bite. By cultivating a mindful approach to eating, endomorphs can better regulate their appetite, improve digestion, and support metabolic health.

4. Regular Evaluation: Regularly evaluate progress and reassess goals to ensure continued growth and improvement. This may involve revisiting meal plans, adjusting workout routines, and seeking support from health professionals as needed.

5. Community and Support: Surround yourself with a supportive community of like-minded individuals who share similar health and fitness goals. Whether it's joining a fitness group, participating in online communities, or seeking guidance from professionals, having a support system can provide motivation, accountability, and encouragement on your journey to optimal metabolic health.

In conclusion, the Metabolic Confusion Meal Plan for Endomorphs offers a holistic approach to optimizing metabolic health, achieving fitness goals, and embracing a sustainable lifestyle. By implementing the principles discussed and incorporating long-term strategies for metabolic health, endomorphs can unleash their metabolic potential and embark on a lifelong journey of vitality, wellness, and vitality.

Let's continue this journey together, empowering each other to thrive and flourish in our pursuit of optimal metabolic health.